STOPPING BREAST CANCER DIET GUIDE FOR WOMEN AGED OVER 40 YEARS

(Exercise program incorporated)

Cancer Health

Healthy Recipe: Black Bean Chili

This is a fast, delicious meal you can put together in about an hour

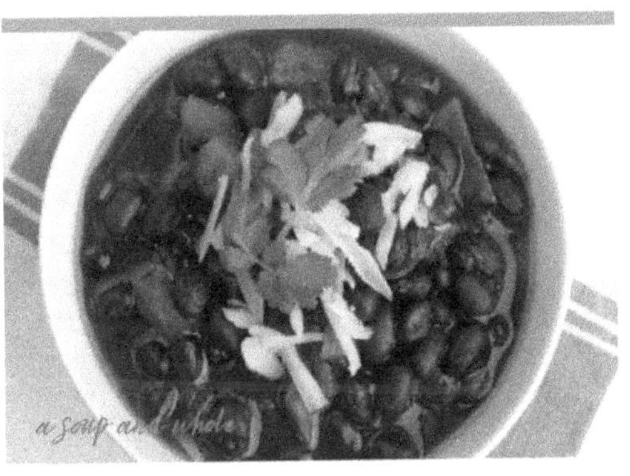

Ultimate Whole Diet Guide for Breast Cancer Prevention and Recurrence with Nutritional Approach.

EPIPHANY HUB PRINTS

STOPPING BREAST CANCER DIET GUIDE FOR WOMEN AGED OVER 40 YEARS

Copyright © [2024] by [EPIPHANY HUB PRINTS]

TABLE OF CONTENTS

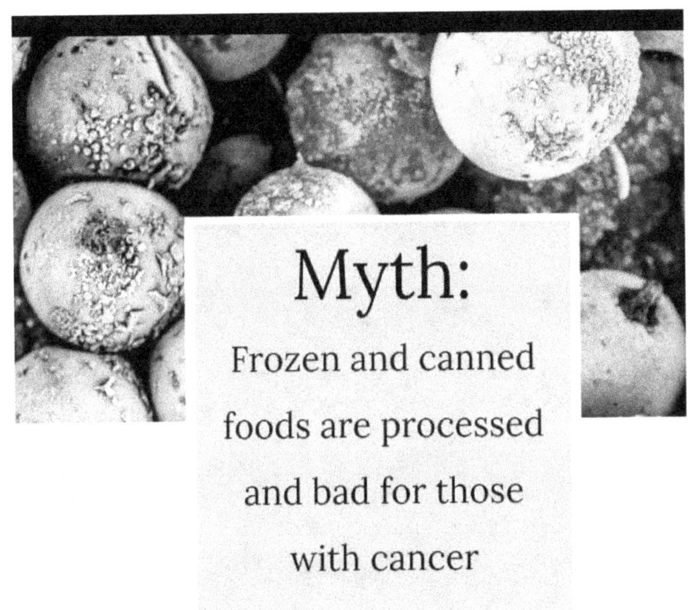

Myth:
Frozen and canned
foods are processed
and bad for those
with cancer

ACT IT

"FIGHT LIKE A WARRIOR, HOPE LIKE A SURVIVOR, AND LOVE LIKE A CONQUEROR."

INTRODUCTION

Greetings from a journey in the kitchen that goes beyond the simple pleasure of cooking to explore the core of health and well-being. Through the pages of this culinary guide, we set out on a mission to empower our communities, our loved ones, and ourselves with the knowledge and skills necessary to fight breast cancer, one delectable recipe at a time.

In the US, around 2,100 men and 240,000 women are diagnosed with breast cancer annually. In the United States, 500 men and 42,000 women pass away from breast cancer annually. Compared to other women, black women die from breast cancer at a higher rate.

Breast cancer is a battle that millions of people throughout the world must fight; it is more than just a diagnosis. However, in the midst of the data and therapies, there is one frequently disregarded ally: the food we eat. Yes, you read correctly: our grocery lists and kitchen cabinets have the power to be powerful allies against this terrible enemy.

In "STOPPING BREAST CANCER DIET GUIDE FOR WOMEN AGED OVER 40 YEARS," we combine the scientific understanding of nutrition with the culinary arts to produce a comprehensive breast cancer defense. In addition to recipes, these sections contain a plethora of information selected by specialists in the culinary arts, nutrition, and oncology.

Every dish, from colorful salads loaded with antioxidants that fight cancer to hearty soups enhanced with herbs that strengthen the immune system, is meticulously designed to satisfy the body and the spirit. However, this cookbook guide serves as a road map for empowerment rather than just a compilation of delicious recipes.

You will find inspiration and direction to help you make important decisions for your health and the health of people you care about, regardless of experience level in the kitchen. Let's work together to turn our kitchens into healing havens where each meal serves as a springboard for a day when breast cancer is not only treated but also preventive.

Come along with us as we set out on a tasty adventure to end breast cancer, one recipe, one mouthful, and one triumph at a time.

CHAPTER ONE

BREAST CANCER AND DIET

Understanding The Link Between Diet and Breast Cancer Risk

Breast cancer continues to be a major global health concern, claiming millions of lives annually. Although there are many factors that lead to the development of breast cancer, new research indicates that nutrition is a major component that can either increase or decrease the risk of the disease.

Knowing this connection enables people to make educated food decisions that may reduce their risk. We explore the complex connection between diet and breast cancer risk in this in-depth guide, providing you with knowledge that will enable you to take preventative action with the "**STOPPING BREAST CANCER DIET GUIDE FOR WOMEN AGED OVER 40 YEARS.**"

Section 1: Exploring the Link Between Diet and Breast Cancer Risk

An overview of breast cancer, including knowledge of its kinds, incidence, and risk factors.

Food's role in the development of breast cancer: describing how dietary factors affect cellular processes linked to cancer formation, inflammation, and hormone homeostasis.

Important food components: investigating how dietary habits, phytochemicals, macro- and micronutrients affect the risk of breast cancer.

The " Stopping Breast Cancer Diet Guide for Women Aged Over 40 Years" introduction: a nutritional strategy supported by research that aims to reduce the risk of breast cancer through diet.

Fundamentals: putting a focus on plant-based sources, nutritious meals, and anti-inflammatory options to foster a healthy eating environment.

Nutritional strategies: Emphasizing particular foods and nutrients, like cruciferous vegetables, berries, omega-3 fatty acids, and vitamin D, that are known to have a preventive impact against breast cancer.

Recipes and meal planning: offering feasible advice on how to incorporate healthy foods into regular meals, along with scrumptious and nourishing recipes designed to promote breast health.

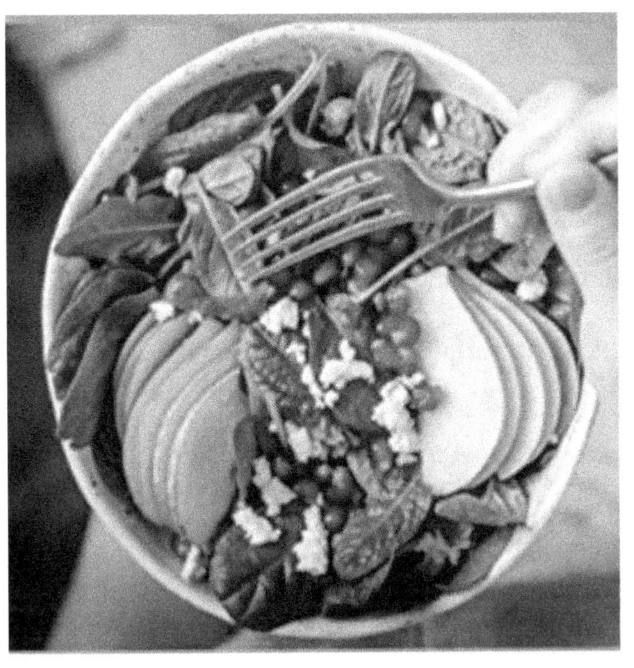

Raising awareness: Talking about the value of education and knowledge in encouraging dietary modifications for the prevention of breast cancer.

Overcoming obstacles: Outlining typical roadblocks to switching to a healthier diet and providing solutions.

Including changes to lifestyle: highlighting the importance of dietary modifications in conjunction with other lifestyle aspects, such as frequent exercise, preserving a healthy weight, and reducing alcohol use.

Resources and community support: Encouraging people to look for advice and encouragement from medical professionals, support groups, and internet communities.

The influence of lobbying enabling people to speak out in favor of legislative initiatives that advance cancer research, provide access to nutrient-dense foods, and increase public understanding of the connection between diet and breast cancer risk.

Highlighting the significance of making proactive dietary decisions in lowering the risk of breast cancer and inspiring readers to get off on their path to ideal breast health with courage and resolve.

Through comprehension of the complex relationship between food and the risk of breast cancer and adoption of the guidelines provided in the " **STOPPING BREAST CANCER DIET GUIDE FOR WOMEN AGED OVER 40 YEARS**," people can proactively mitigate their risk and enhance their general well-being. Never forget that every food decision counts. Let's give ourselves the power to make decisions that promote our health and energy.

Dietary Decisions Are Crucial for Treatment and Prevention

There is a complex relationship between diet and breast cancer. Research has repeatedly demonstrated that eating habits can affect a person's chance of getting breast cancer. For example, diets heavy in sugar, processed foods, and saturated fats have been connected to an increased risk; on the other hand, diets high in whole grains, fruits, vegetables, and lean proteins have been linked to a decreased risk.

Prevention through Nutrition:

Eating a balanced diet and staying at a healthy weight are important aspects in preventing breast cancer. The " Stopping Breast Cancer Diet Guide for Women Aged Over 40 Years " places a strong emphasis on including foods high in antioxidants, vitamins, and minerals, as well as nutrient density. In addition to promoting general health, these foods strengthen the body's defenses against malignant cells.

In addition, the cooking guide promotes the intake of foods high in phytochemicals, which have been demonstrated to have anti-cancer qualities, like cruciferous vegetables, berries, and green tea. People can alter the environment in their bodies to make it less favorable for cancer to develop by switching to a plant-based diet that is supplemented with lean proteins and healthy fats.

Management and Supportive Nutrition:

Diet is a major factor in treatment results and general health for individuals who have been diagnosed with breast cancer. A few dietary practices can enhance the body's natural healing and recovery processes while reducing the negative effects of therapies like radiation and chemotherapy.

Recipes from the " **STOPPING BREAST CANCER DIET GUIDE FOR WOMEN AGED OVER 40 YEARS**" are adapted to meet the unique dietary requirements of cancer patients. The main goal of these recipes is to supply enough nutrients to boost immunity, fight exhaustion, and lessen inflammation. The cookbook also stresses the significance of eating foods that support gut health and being properly hydrated, since gut microbiota has been connected to the prevention and treatment of cancer.

Giving People Knowledge and Recipes: The " **STOPPING BREAST CANCER DIET GUIDE FOR WOMEN AGED OVER 40 YEARS**" is a comprehensive resource that teaches people about the science underlying nutrition and breast cancer, in addition to offering recipes. People are more equipped to make decisions regarding their health and well-being when they are aware of how dietary choices affect cancer risk and progression.

The cooking guide also highlights the significance of dietary modifications together with lifestyle aspects like consistent exercise, stress reduction, and enough sleep for the best prevention and treatment of breast cancer.

Dietary decisions have a big impact on the battle against breast cancer. People can lower their risk of breast cancer and improve their general health by embracing a diet high in whole, nutrient-dense foods and adopting healthy lifestyle practices.

The "Stopping Breast Cancer Diet Guide for Women Aged Over 40 Years" is an invaluable resource in this effort, providing scrumptious dishes and inspiring information to enable people to make decisions that will lead to a healthier future.

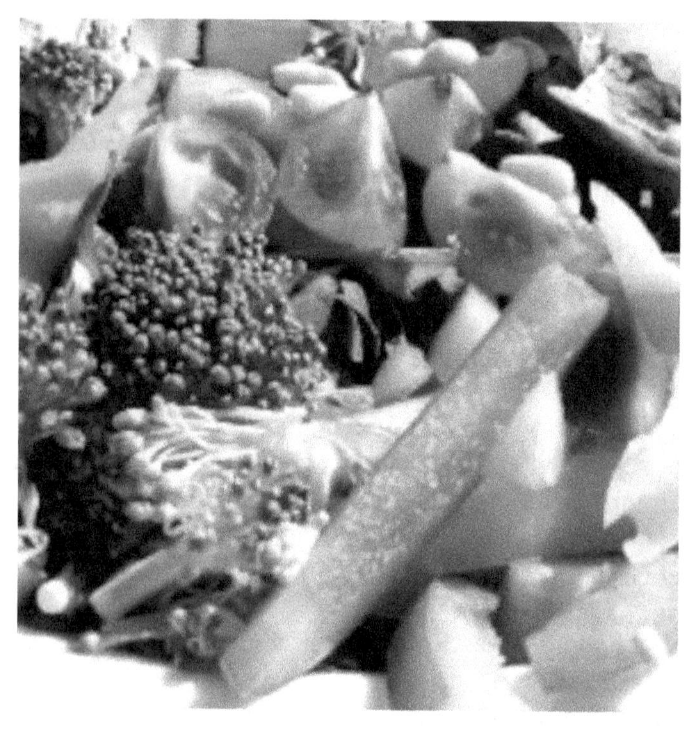

CHAPTER TWO

THE ROLE OF NUTRITION IN BREAST CANCER PREVENTION

Breast cancer is a global health concern that affects millions of people. Although genetics do play a part, nutrition and other lifestyle choices are becoming more and more acknowledged as important influences on breast health. Our ability to incorporate vital nutrients that support good breast health into our diets is the first step on the quest to prevent breast cancer.

We explore the significance of essential nutrients and their influence on breast health in this synopsis, as indicated by the "STOPPING BREAST CANCER DIET GUIDE FOR WOMEN AGED OVER 40 YEARS."

Vitamin D:

Vitamin D, sometimes known as the "sunshine vitamin," is essential for preserving breast health. Sufficient amounts of vitamin D have been linked in research to a lower risk of breast cancer. This vitamin may prevent the formation of malignant cells by regulating cellular growth and bolstering the immune system. Sunlight exposure, supplements, fortified dairy products, and fatty seafood like salmon and mackerel are good sources of vitamin D.

Antioxidants:

Strong substances called antioxidants shield cells against oxidative stress brought on by free radicals, unstable chemicals associated with the onset of cancer. Including foods high in antioxidants in your diet can help combat free radical damage and lower your chance of developing breast cancer. Antioxidants are abundant in colorful fruits and vegetables, including bell peppers, tomatoes, spinach, and berries. These anti-cancer ingredients are also abundant in dark chocolate, almonds, seeds, and green tea.

Omega-3 Fatty Acids:

These important fats have anti-inflammatory qualities that promote breast health as well as general wellness. According to studies, omega-3 fatty acids may stop tumor growth and lower the chance of breast cancer returning. Omega-3s can be found in large quantities in fatty fish like salmon, trout, and sardines as well as in plant-based foods like walnuts, chia seeds, and flaxseeds.

Cruciferous Vegetables:

Brussels sprouts, broccoli, cauliflower, kale, and other cruciferous vegetables have special substances called glucosinolates. Glucosinolates are broken down during digestion to yield bioactive compounds with anti-cancer characteristics. By decreasing inflammation and regulating estrogen metabolism, these veggies may help lessen the risk of breast cancer.

Fiber:

Consuming a diet high in fiber can help with digestion and lower the risk of developing chronic illnesses like breast cancer, among other health benefits. Fiber aids in the body's excretion of estrogen, which helps to maintain healthy levels of the hormone. Vegetables, fruits, whole grains, and legumes are all great sources of dietary fiber that can help maintain good breast health.

Phytoestrogens:

Plant-based substances called phytoestrogens function similarly to estrogen in the body. By occupying estrogen receptors and regulating hormone levels, phytoestrogens may have preventive effects even when excessive estrogen exposure is associated with a higher risk of breast cancer. Whole grains, flaxseeds, and sesame seeds are excellent sources of phytoestrogens, as are soy products like tofu, tempeh, and edamame.

You may significantly lower your risk of breast cancer and promote breast health by including these essential nutrients in your diet. To fully utilize the nutritional potential of these ingredients in tasty and satisfying meals, the "Stopping

Breast Cancer Diet Guide for Women Aged Over 40 Years"
provides a plethora of dish ideas and culinary inspiration.

You may protect your breast health and general health by
making a diet high in vitamin D, antioxidants, omega-3 fatty
acids, cruciferous vegetables, fiber, and phytoestrogens a
priority. Always keep in mind that every meal is a chance to
help your body reach its full potential in terms of health and
energy.

Dietary Guidelines for Reducing Breast Cancer Risk

Although there are other factors including genetics involved,
new research indicates that dietary decisions can have a
major impact on the risk of breast cancer. The Stopping
Breast Cancer Diet Guide for Women Aged Over 40 Years
provides a thorough roadmap for selecting foods that lower
this risk. Let's explore the key dietary recommendations for
lowering the risk of breast cancer and how this cookbook
might be a useful tool.

Accept a Diet Based on Plants:

Throughout your meals, include a range of fruits, vegetables,
whole grains, and legumes.
Try to consume five servings or more of fruits and
vegetables each day.
Select vibrant produce that is high in antioxidants, like
tomatoes, leafy greens, and berries.

Limit Red and Processed Meats:

Limit your intake of red meats, such as lamb, hog, and beef.
Reduce your consumption of processed meats like sausage, bacon, and deli meats.
As an alternative, choose lean protein sources including fish, poultry, tofu, and lentils.

Opt for Healthy Fats:

Select foods like avocados, almonds, seeds, and olive oil that are high in healthful fats.
Cut back on the saturated fats in cheese, butter, and fatty meats.
Avert trans fats, which are frequently included in processed and fried foods.

Moderate Alcohol Consumption:

Women should only have one drink of alcohol per day. For celebratory events, think about options like fruit-flavored sparkling water.

Increase Fiber Intake:

Add foods high in fiber, such as fruits, vegetables, whole grains, beans, and lentils.
To support digestive health and lower the risk of cancer, try to consume at least 25–30 grams of fiber per day.

Be Mindful of Portion Sizes:

To control calorie consumption and keep a healthy weight, practice portion management.
To avoid overindulging, use smaller plates and steer clear of excessive servings.

Stay Hydrated:

Stay hydrated and promote general health throughout the day by drinking lots of water.
Drink less sugary drinks and more water, herbal tea, or infused water.

Include Spices and Herbs that Fight Cancer:

Try experimenting with anti-inflammatory and antioxidant-rich herbs and spices such as cinnamon, ginger, garlic, and turmeric.

Opt for whole foods rather than processed foods.

Choose minimally processed, unprocessed foods over those that are packed and processed.
Examine product labels and steer clear of items heavy in toxic additives, processed grains, and added sugars.

Seek Support and Resources:

Make use of resources such as the Stopping Breast Cancer Diet Guide for Women Aged Over 40 Years for meal planning, recipes, and advice specific to lowering the risk of breast cancer through diet. For individualized counsel, think about attending support groups or consulting a certified dietitian with expertise in oncology nutrition.

Succintly, making dietary choices that lower the risk of breast cancer is a proactive and empowering action that each and every person can perform. Through adherence to these dietary recommendations and utilization of tools such as the Stopping Breast Cancer Diet Guide for Women Aged Over 40 Years, people can develop a nutritious and anti-cancer diet.

Recall that minor adjustments can have a big effects on long-term health and wellbeing. Let's embrace the role that nutrition plays in lowering the risk of breast cancer and enhancing general health and energy.

TOP ANTI-CANCER FOODS

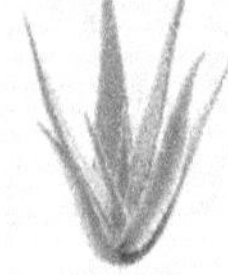

Aloe Vera

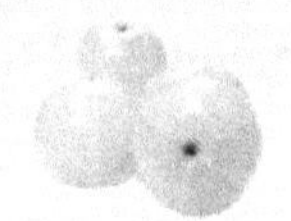

Amla Berries

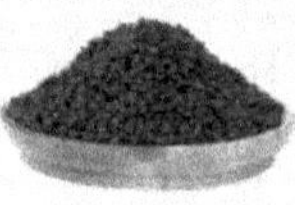

Nigella Seeds

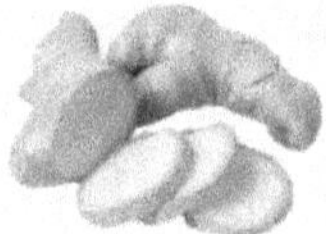

GInger

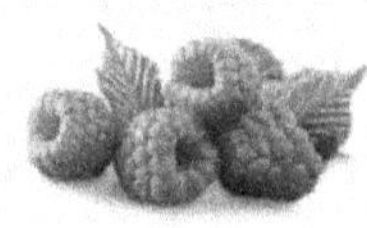

Raspberries

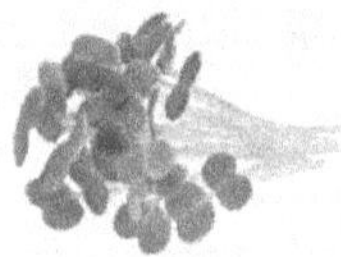

Sprouts

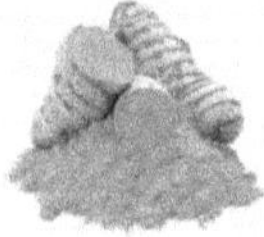

Turmeric

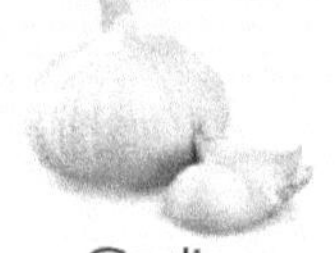

Garlic

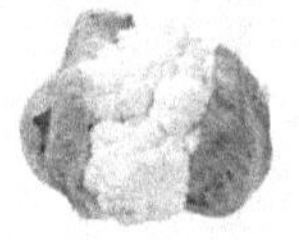

Cauliflower

@transformativehealthcoach

CHAPTER THREE

PLANT-BASED DIET AND BREAST CANCER

Evidence indicates that food plays a critical role in lowering the chance of getting breast cancer, even though not all occurrences of the illness are avoidable. A diet high in plant-based foods, such as fruits, vegetables, whole grains, legumes, nuts, and seeds, may help reduce the risk of breast cancer, according to several studies.

Principal Advantages of a Plant-Based Diet for Breast Health:

A Plant-Based Diet Has a Number of Possible Benefits for Managing and Preventing Breast Cancer:

Rich in Antioxidants: Rich in antioxidants, which assist the body in scavenging dangerous free radicals, are fruits, vegetables, nuts, seeds, and whole grains. Free radicals have the ability to harm cells and promote the growth of cancer. Vitamins C and E, beta-carotene, selenium, and other antioxidants present in plant-based diets may help lower the risk of breast cancer.

Rich in phytochemicals: Numerous phytonutrients, such as flavonoids, phenolic acids, and carotenoids, which have anti-inflammatory and anticancer characteristics, can be found in plant-based diets. These substances might lessen the chance of a breast cancer recurrence and decrease the proliferation of cancer cells.

Fiber Content: Diets based mostly on plants tend to be high in fiber, which supports healthy digestion and aids in hormone regulation. Because high-fiber diets help the body rid itself of excess estrogen, which can feed hormone-sensitive breast cancers, they have been linked to a lower risk of breast cancer.

Naturally low in saturated fat: Saturated fat is mostly found in animal products and is absent from plant-based diets. An elevated risk of breast cancer has been associated with high intake of saturated fat, particularly in postmenopausal women. Selecting fats from plants, such as olive oil, avocados, nuts, and seeds, can help reduce the amount of saturated fat consumed overall.

Weight management: Diets high in plant-based foods tend to be higher in nutrient density and lower in calories than diets high in animal products. Since extra body fat, particularly around the waist, is linked to an increased risk of postmenopausal breast cancer, maintaining a healthy weight is crucial for lowering the risk of breast cancer.

Hormonal Balance: Phytoestrogens, or plant substances that mimic the actions of estrogen in the body, are present in several plant foods, such as flaxseeds and soybeans. These foods can help balance hormone levels and lower the risk of hormone receptor-positive breast cancer when consumed in moderation.

Encouragement of Healthy Lifestyle Habits: Eating a plant-based diet frequently goes hand in hand with other healthy lifestyle decisions including getting regular exercise, limiting alcohol intake, and quitting smoking. When these lifestyle variables are combined, the risk of breast cancer can be further decreased, and general health and wellbeing can be enhanced.

Although there are many potential advantages to a plant-based diet for managing and preventing breast cancer, it's crucial to speak with a medical professional or registered dietitian to ensure adequate nutrition and individualized dietary recommendations based on a person's health status and medical history.

A complete strategy to prevent and treat breast cancer should also include lifestyle changes, adequate medical care, and routine tests. This includes including a plant-based diet into this strategy

Incorporating Fruits, Vegetables, And Plant Proteins into Your Meals

Along with being good for your health, include fruits, veggies, and plant proteins in your meals also gives your diet some flavor and diversity. The following advice will help you include these wholesome ingredients with ease:

Begin with a Colorful Base: **Base** your meals on an assortment of vibrant fruits and vegetables. Add colorful vegetables like bell peppers, carrots, and tomatoes, as well as a variety of greens like spinach, kale, and broccoli. This not only adds visual appeal to your dish but also guarantees that you're getting a variety of vitamins, minerals, and antioxidants.

Try a Variety of Cooking Techniques: **To** bring out the flavors and textures of your veggies, try roasting, grilling, steaming, or sautéing them. You may add intriguing flavor to even the most basic veggies by experimenting with cooking techniques.

Blend Them in: **Add** fruits and veggies to smoothies, soups, and sauces to make them a part of your meals. For instance, pureed butternut squash can be used to make a creamy spaghetti sauce, or for an added nutritional boost, blend spinach and berries into your morning smoothie.

Replace Meat with Plant Proteins: **You** can incorporate plant-based protein sources like tofu, tempeh, legumes (beans, lentils, and chickpeas), quinoa, or seitan into your meals in place of some or all of the meat. These choices are abundant in fiber and other necessary nutrients, in addition to being high in protein.

Bring Ingenuity to Your Salads: **You** don't have to eat boring salads! To make tasty and filling salads, toss in a variety of fruits, nuts, seeds, and even cooked grains like farro or quinoa. For extra taste, garnish them with creamy avocado-based sauces or homemade vinaigrettes.

Snack Wisely: Choose whole fruits, veggies with hummus or nut butter, or a handful of nuts and seeds as your snack of choice rather than processed foods. Having wholesome snacks on hand facilitates making nutrient-dense decisions all day long.

Plan Ahead: Including more fruits, veggies, and plant-based proteins in your meals can be achieved via meal planning and preparation. Every week, set aside some time to plan your snacks and meals. To speed up the cooking process, prepare items ahead of time.

Accept Seasonal Produce: Eating fruits and vegetables in season guarantees that you're consuming the freshest and tastiest produce possible while also helping your community's farmers. To find seasonal treasures, check out farmers' markets or sign up for a community-supported agriculture (CSA) program.

You'll find a world of delectable and fulfilling culinary choices as well as enhance your general health by including more fruits, veggies, and plant proteins in your meals. Try with various ingredients and cooking methods to see what suits you the best, and have fun as you move toward a diet that is more plant-based!

The Power of Fruits in Your Diet:

Note:

Look into different fruits that are especially good for preventing breast cancer, like apples, avocado, berries, and citrus fruits.
Give inventive ideas for using fruits into salads, smoothies, and fruit-based treats.
Stress how important it is to select whole fruits rather than processed ones in order to get the most nutritional value.

Harnessing the Nutritional Value of Vegetables:

Using the nutritional value of vegetables for breast cancer entails including a range of nutrient-rich vegetables in your diet to enhance general health, maybe lower your chance of acquiring breast cancer, or assist in the treatment process.

Here's how to accomplish it:

Put an Emphasis on a Colorful Variety: Try to choose vegetables that range in hue from light to dark. Vegetables with different colors have different antioxidant, vitamin, and mineral contents that have different health advantages. For instance, orange veggies like carrots and sweet potatoes are high in beta-carotene, while dark leafy greens like spinach and kale are rich in folate.

Cruciferous Vegetables: Cruciferous vegetables, which include cabbage, Brussels sprouts, cauliflower, and broccoli, are especially helpful in preventing breast cancer. They contain substances known as glucosinolates, which have been demonstrated to possess anti-cancer qualities. Sulforaphane, a substance that may aid in halting the growth of breast cancer cells, is also present in these veggies.

Integrate Onions and Garlic: As members of the Allium vegetable family, onions and garlic contain sulfur compounds that may lower the risk of cancer. Lower incidence of breast cancer and other cancers have been associated with certain veggies. To take advantage of their potential benefits, include them in your meals on a regular basis, either raw or cooked.

Tomatoes and Bell Peppers: Packed with antioxidants like vitamin C and lycopene, tomatoes and bell peppers may help prevent breast cancer. Particularly lycopene has been researched for its anti-cancer effects. Savor them raw in salads, sautéed in sauces, or roasted to serve as an accompaniment.

Leafy Greens: Rich in nutrients, leafy greens like Swiss chard, spinach, and kale are superfoods. They are abundant in antioxidants, vitamins, and minerals that promote general health and may lower the incidence of breast cancer. You may sauté them as a side dish or add them to soups, salads, and smoothies.

Herbs and Spices: Due to their strong anti-inflammatory and antioxidant qualities, herbs and spices like cinnamon, ginger, and turmeric may help prevent breast cancer. Specifically, curcumin, found in turmeric, has being researched for possible anti-cancer properties. Use these spices and herbs in your food to enhance flavor and nutritional value.

Reduce Processed meals: In addition to concentrating on eating more nutrient-dense veggies, you should also reduce processed meals, sugary snacks, and refined carbohydrates. These foods can cause oxidative stress and inflammation in the body, and they have been linked to an increased risk of breast cancer.

Speak with a Registered Dietitian: If you are receiving treatment for breast cancer or have questions about a particular diet, you should think about speaking with a registered dietitian who specializes in oncology nutrition. They may offer customized advice based on your particular requirements and assist you in making the best dietary choices for your general health and wellbeing.

A nutritious diet that includes a wide range of nutrient-rich vegetables is crucial for promoting overall wellbeing and maybe lowering the risk of breast cancer. For best results, remember to incorporate a balanced diet, frequent exercise, and other healthful lifestyle choices.

Plant Proteins: Building Blocks of a Healthy Diet:

Introduce protein options derived from plants, such as quinoa, tofu, tempeh, and lentils.

Talk about the advantages of using plant-based proteins in place of animal proteins for cancer prevention and general wellness.
Provide scrumptious and nutrient-dense meal ideas and recipes that highlight the adaptability of plant proteins.

Useful Hints for Including Plant-Based Foods in Your Everyday Diet:

Provide meal planning techniques to guarantee a consumption of fruits, vegetables, and plant-based proteins that is balanced.

For individuals who are used to eating a lot of meat, offer strategies for a gradual shift to a more plant-based diet. Give advice on how to choose nutrient-dense, whole foods and how to read food labels.

Healthy Recipe: Quinoa Breakfast Porridge

Feel free to use any topping you'd like

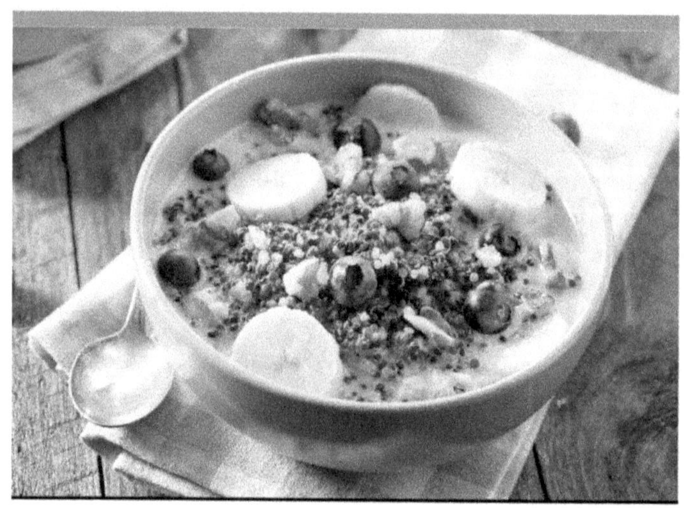

CHAPTER FOUR

ANTI-INFLAMMATORY FOODS FOR BREAST HEALTH

Understanding Inflammation and Its Role in Breast Cancer

Chronic inflammation in breast cancer has been linked to the disease from its onset to its metastases. A microenvironment that is created by inflammatory cells and chemicals in breast tissue encourages the growth, invasion, and angiogenesis (the development of new blood vessels to nourish tumors) of cancer cells. Furthermore, inflammation might exacerbate treatment resistance and impair a patient's overall prognosis in cases of breast cancer.

Key Dietary Factors in Inflammation and Breast Cancer:

An important factor in controlling inflammation in the body is diet. It has been demonstrated that several foods and nutrients can increase or decrease inflammation, which affects the risk of breast cancer. The following dietary considerations are listed:

Anti-inflammatory Foods:

Consume an abundance of fruits, vegetables, whole grains, nuts, seeds, and fatty fish that is high in omega-3 fatty acids as anti-inflammatory foods. These foods can help reduce inflammation because they include anti-inflammatory and antioxidant properties.

Omega-3 Fatty Acids:

Rich in flaxseeds, chia seeds, walnuts, and fatty fish (salmon, mackerel, and sardines), omega-3 fatty acids have strong anti-inflammatory qualities. Frequent consumption may help lessen the risk of breast cancer and minimize inflammation.

Antioxidants:

Rich in vitamins C and E, beta-carotene, and flavonoids, colorful fruits and vegetables like berries, spinach, kale, and tomatoes also contain a lot of antioxidants. Antioxidants aid in the reduction of damage caused by inflammation and the neutralization of free radicals.

Good Fats:

Choose for healthy fats that come from nuts, avocados, and olive oil. These foods contain monounsaturated and polyunsaturated fatty acids, also known as omega-6 fatty acids. When ingested in moderation, these fats can help control inflammation.

Eat Less Inflammatory Foods:

Reduce your consumption of processed meals, sugary snacks, red and processed meats, refined carbohydrates, and foods high in trans fats. These foods may raise the risk of breast cancer and have been linked to inflammation.

Such as quercetin (found in onions and apples), resveratrol (found in grapes and red wine), and curcumin (found in turmeric). These substances have anti-inflammatory and anti-tumor effects.

Including Foods and Spices That Reduce Inflammation in Your Diet

You can assist lower inflammation in the body and possibly minimize your risk of breast cancer by include anti-inflammatory foods and spices in your diet.

Key Anti-Inflammatory Foods and Spices:

Turmeric: The active ingredient in turmeric, curcumin, has strong anti-inflammatory effects. Turmeric can help lower inflammation and improve general health when added to food or taken as supplements.

Berries: Rich in antioxidants and flavonoids, which have anti-inflammatory properties, blueberries, strawberries, and raspberries are berries. Including a range of berries in your diet has many health advantages, one of which being the reduction of inflammation.

Fatty Fish: Rich in omega-3 fatty acids, which have anti-inflammatory qualities, salmon, mackerel, and sardines are great sources of this nutrient. Regularly eating fatty fish can promote breast health and reduce inflammation.

Leafy Greens: Rich in vitamins, minerals, and phytonutrients that help lower inflammation in the body are spinach, kale, and Swiss chard. To promote general health, try to incorporate leafy greens into your meals on a daily basis.

Ginger: The bioactive molecule gingerol, which has potent anti-inflammatory and antioxidant qualities, is found in ginger. Drinking ginger tea or incorporating fresh ginger into your food can help reduce inflammation and support breast health.

Garlic: Studies have indicated that sulfur compounds found in garlic can reduce inflammation. Adding garlic to your food can improve its flavor and offer several health advantages, such as lowering inflammation.

Useful Hints for Including Anti-Inflammatory Spices and Foods:

Have a healthy breakfast that includes anti-inflammatory foods like nuts, Greek yogurt, and berries to start your day. Add turmeric to smoothies, curries, stews, and soups to include it into your food.

Eat little amounts of fresh produce, nuts, and fruits throughout the day to reduce inflammation. At least twice a week, incorporate fatty fish into your diet by grilling, roasting, or broiling it for a tasty and nutritious dinner.

Try experimenting with various herbs and spices, like garlic, ginger, cinnamon, and rosemary, to give your food taste and anti-inflammatory properties.

Replace refined grains with whole grains, such as quinoa, brown rice, and oats; these foods are higher in nutrients and fiber and can help lower inflammation.

Refined carbs, sugary snacks, and processed foods should be consumed in moderation as they might aggravate inflammation in the body.

Including foods and spices high in anti-inflammatory properties in your diet can help to promote breast health and lower your risk of breast cancer. You may use nutrition to enhance general well-being and reduce inflammation in your body by heeding the helpful advice in this book and making thoughtful dietary choices.

Before making any big dietary changes, always get advice from a medical expert or a certified dietician, particularly if you have any pre-existing medical illnesses or concerns. You can take proactive measures to avoid breast cancer and live a longer, healthier life with a nutritious, well-balanced diet.

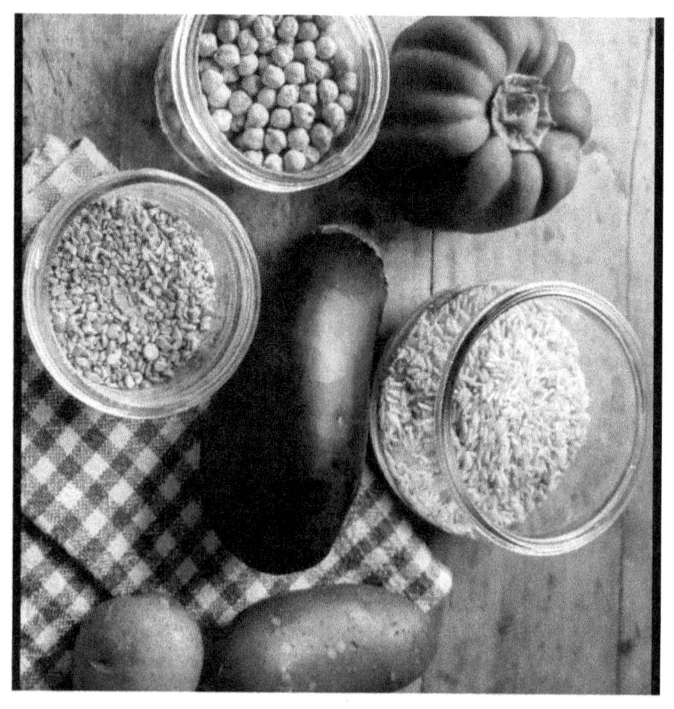

CHAPTER FIVE

HEALTHY FATS AND BREAST CANCER RISK

Differentiating Between Healthy and Unhealthy Fats

Healthy Fats:

Healthy fats include monounsaturated and polyunsaturated fats, which are frequently found in foods like avocados, nuts, seeds, and fatty fish.

It is well recognized that these fats lower cholesterol, promote heart health, and facilitate the absorption of fat-soluble vitamins.
According to studies, eating more of these fats may help lessen inflammation and the chance of developing several malignancies, including breast cancer.

Unhealthy Fats:

Trans fats and saturated fats are regarded as harmful fats. Animal goods like red meat, butter, and cheese, as well as some plant-based oils like coconut and palm oil, are the main sources of saturated fats.

Trans fats are especially dangerous because they elevate LDL cholesterol levels, increase the risk of heart disease, and cause inflammation. They are frequently found in processed and fried meals.

A growing body of research indicates that diets heavy in trans and saturated fats may also raise the risk of breast cancer.

Healthy Fats and Breast Cancer Risk:

A lower risk of breast cancer may be linked to diets high in monounsaturated and polyunsaturated fats, according to research.
These fats help fight oxidative stress and inflammation, two factors that are connected to the development of cancer. They also include antioxidants and anti-inflammatory qualities.
The potential preventive effects of omega-3 fatty acids against breast cancer have been the subject of specific research. Sardines and other fatty fish are high in omega-3 fatty acids.

Unhealthy Fats and Breast Cancer Risk:

On the other hand, diets heavy in trans and saturated fats may raise the risk of breast cancer.

Breast cancer cells may proliferate as a result of inflammation and estrogen production that is encouraged by saturated fats.

Studies on animals have demonstrated that trans fats disrupt hormone balance and encourage the formation of tumors; however, further investigation is required to confirm a direct connection in people.

Practical Dietary Tips:

Select plant-based fat sources over animal-based saturated fats, such as those found in avocados, nuts, seeds, and olive oil.

Regularly include fatty fish that is high in omega-3 fatty acids in your diet.

Eat fewer processed and fried foods that are high in trans fats.

Carefully read food labels and choose goods that have the fewest amount of trans and saturated fats.

Aim for a diet rich in nutrients and well-balanced to improve general health and lower the risk of breast cancer.

Making educated dietary decisions can significantly lower the risk of breast cancer, even if no one food or vitamin will ensure prevention.

Selecting Healthy Fat Sources to Lower The Risk Of Breast Cancer

Not every fat is made equally. Healthy fats are crucial for preserving optimum health, even though trans and saturated fats are linked to negative health outcomes like obesity and cardiovascular disorders.

Good fats, such as polyunsaturated and monounsaturated fats, provide many health advantages, such as lowering inflammation, promoting heart health, and enhancing brain function. Furthermore, a lower risk of breast cancer has been associated with specific types of good fats.

Choosing Sources of Healthy Fats:

Fatty Fish: Omega-3 fatty acids, a kind of polyunsaturated fat with anti-inflammatory qualities, are abundant in fatty fish, including salmon, mackerel, and sardines. According to studies, by lowering inflammation in breast tissue and preventing tumor formation, omega-3 fatty acids may help lower the risk of breast cancer.

Nuts and Seeds: Rich sources of good fats, especially omega-3 and monounsaturated fats, include almonds, walnuts, flaxseeds, and chia seeds. A small amount of good fats and other vital nutrients can be greatly increased by include a handful of nuts or seeds in your diet on a regular basis. This can improve general health and possibly lower your risk of breast cancer.

Avocado: Packed with nutrients, avocados are especially high in oleic acid and other monounsaturated fats. Aside from giving foods a richer, more flavorful texture, avocados are a good source of healthful fats that may help reduce your risk of breast cancer.

Olive Oil: Extra virgin olive oil is highly valued for its profusion of monounsaturated fats and antioxidant components, making it a mainstay of the Mediterranean diet. Frequent use of olive oil has been linked to a lower risk of breast cancer among other illnesses.

Coconut Oil: Although it is a contentious substance, coconut oil has medium-chain triglycerides (MCTs), which may have health advantages. Despite the paucity of data on the direct effects of coconut oil on the incidence of breast cancer, a balanced diet moderately containing coconut oil.

Making informed choices about the fats you eat is one of the most significant things you can do to reduce your risk of breast cancer and enhance your overall health. Eating more avocado, nuts, seeds, fatty fish, olive oil, and coconut oil—foods high in healthy fats—will fuel your body and may lower your risk of breast cancer.

Did you know?

An anti-inflammatory diet may not only reduce cancer risk but is also associated with reduced mortality risk among breast cancer survivors.

CHAPTER SIX
PHYTONUTRIENTS AND BREAST CANCER PROTECTION

Exploring The Role of Phytonutrients in Cancer Prevention

Phytochemicals, another name for phytonutrients, are substances that are present in plants that have been proved to provide health advantages over just food. The vivid hues, tastes, and scents of fruits, vegetables, herbs, and spices are brought about by these bioactive substances. Among the several types of phytonutrients include glucosinolates, flavonoids, carotenoids, and polyphenols.

Phytonutrients' Anti-Cancer Properties: Studies show that phytonutrients have strong anti-inflammatory, antioxidant, and anticancer effects. They assist the body's defense processes naturally, lessen inflammation, control cell growth, and neutralize dangerous free radicals. Numerous scholarly investigations have emphasized the function of phytonutrients in impeding the proliferation and dissemination of cancerous cells, particularly those connected to breast cancer.

Specific Phytonutrients and Breast Cancer Prevention:

Flavonoids: Are plentiful in fruits, vegetables, tea, red wine, and other foods. Studies have linked flavonoids to a lower risk of breast cancer. Two prominent examples of flavonoids having anti-cancer qualities are quercetin, which is present in apples and onions, and catechins, which are prevalent in green tea.

Carotenoids: These pigments are responsible for the vivid colors of fruits and vegetables. Beta-carotene (found in carrots, sweet potatoes, and spinach) and lycopene (found in abundance in tomatoes) are two carotenoids that have been associated with a decreased risk of breast cancer.

Polyphenols: Found in a wide range of plant foods, polyphenols have potent antioxidant properties. Two well-researched polyphenols with possible anti-cancer properties include resveratrol, which is found in berries and grapes, and epigallocatechin gallate (EGCG), which is found in green tea.

Cruciferous Vegetables: Broccoli, cauliflower, kale, and Brussels sprouts are examples of vegetables high in glucosinolates, sulfur-containing substances that may lessen the risk of breast cancer. These veggies also contain sulforaphane, which has been shown in numerous studies to have anti-cancer properties.

Including colorful fruits, veggies, and herbs to reap the advantages of phytonutrients

Phytonutrients, sometimes referred to as phytochemicals, are substances that naturally exist in plants. These substances are responsible for the vivid hues and unique tastes of fruits, vegetables, and herbs. More significantly, they provide a host of health advantages, such as anti-inflammatory and antioxidant qualities that are essential in lowering the risk of chronic illnesses like cancer.

Colorful Fruits and Phytonutrient Benefits:

Red and Pink: Lycopene is a potent antioxidant that may lower the risk of breast cancer. Fruits and vegetables that are high in this compound include tomatoes, strawberries, watermelon, and pink grapefruit. Lycopene prevents the growth of cancer cells and aids in the neutralization of free radicals.

Orange and Yellow: Research has linked carotenoids, such as beta-carotene from squash, sweet potatoes, and carrots, to a decreased risk of breast cancer. These substances help prevent cancer by boosting immunological function in addition to offering antioxidant defense.

Green: Rich in lutein, zeaxanthin, and chlorophyll, leafy greens like broccoli, spinach, and kale have been associated with a lower risk of breast cancer. These nutrients aid in the body's detoxification procedures and provide protection against oxidative stress.

Blue and purple: Anthocyanins, which are present in purple grapes, blackberries, and blueberries, have strong anti-inflammatory and antioxidant qualities. They may prevent cancer cells from proliferating and aid in the defense of cells against harm.

Incorporating Colorful Foods into Your Diet:

A colorful smoothie made with leafy greens and a range of colorful fruits is a great way to start the day. Throughout the day, nibble on a rainbow of fresh fruits and vegetables.

Include vibrant salads in your meals that feature a variety of fruits, veggies, and herbs.

Try experimenting with vibrant spices and herbs like cilantro, ginger, and turmeric to give your food more taste and health benefits from phytonutrients.

Colorful substitutes for processed foods include dried fruits, mixed nuts, and seeds.

Utilizing a diet abundant in vibrant fruits, vegetables, and herbs, you can use the potential of phytonutrients to mitigate your chances of developing breast cancer. These plant-based diets contain a wide range of phytochemicals that combine to support general health and wellbeing in addition to providing vital vitamins and minerals. Transform each meal into a vibrant celebration of life and energy, and take preventative measures to avoid breast cancer.

CHAPTER SEVEN

LIMITING PROCESSED FOODS AND SUGAR

Understanding The Impact of Processed Foods and Sugar On Breast Health

High concentrations of chemicals, preservatives, refined sugars, and harmful fats are characteristics of processed foods. Frequent use of these foods has been linked to a number of health problems, such as diabetes, heart disease, and obesity.

Furthermore, a number of studies have shown a link between eating processed foods and a higher risk of breast cancer. These foods frequently include toxic substances that can upset hormonal balance and cause nutritional deficiencies, which may encourage the growth of malignant cells in breast tissue.

Understanding the Role of Sugar in Breast Health:

It has long been known that consuming too much sugar can exacerbate a number of health issues, including diabetes and obesity. Less is known about its effects on breast health, though. Consuming large amounts of sugar can increase insulin resistance and insulin levels, which can encourage the growth and division of cancer cells, including those found in breast tissue.

Moreover, consuming sugar has been connected to chronic inflammation, which is a recognized risk factor for the development of breast cancer. Diets high in sugar also frequently lack important nutrients, which further impairs general health and immune system performance.

Navigating Dietary Choices for Breast Health:

To preserve optimum breast health and lower the risk of breast cancer, mindful eating is essential. The following are some doable actions that people can take:

Give whole, nutrient-dense foods a priority: Choose whole foods including whole grains, fruits, veggies, lean meats, and healthy fats. Essential vitamins, minerals, and antioxidants found in these foods promote general health and may offer some protection against breast cancer.

Reduce Your Consumption of Processed meals and Added Sugars: Cut back on your intake of soda, sugary drinks, sugary snacks, and processed meals. Instead, study food labels to find hidden sugars in packaged goods and use natural sweeteners like honey or maple syrup sparingly.

Accept a Balanced Diet: Make an effort to eat a balanced diet that contains the range of nutrients required to keep your health at its best. Include entire grains, lean meats, vibrant fruits and veggies, and healthy fats in your meals.

Remain Hydrated: Drink mostly water or herbal teas instead of sugary drinks and large amounts of caffeine, which can upset your hormone balance and cause inflammation.

Practice Mindful Eating: Eat consciously by being aware of your hunger cues, controlling your portion sizes, and taking time to appreciate every bite. This can encourage a positive relationship with food and help avoid overindulging.

Dietary decisions are crucial for preserving breast health and lowering the chance of breast cancer, even if genetics and other variables also increase the risk of breast cancer. A balanced diet, a reduction in processed foods and added sugars, and a focus on whole, nutrient-dense foods can empower people to take charge of their health and reduce their risk of breast cancer. A potent weapon in the fight against breast cancer is making educated food decisions that promote long-term health and energy.

Tips for Reducing Consumption of Processed Foods and Added Sugars

Fortunately, the consumption of these dangerous substances can be greatly decreased, possibly lowering the risk of breast cancer, by implementing small dietary adjustments. Here are five practical methods to help you cut back on added sugars and processed foods in your diet.

An Overlooked Food in a Plant-Based Diet for Cancer Prevention

Many people are unfamiliar with, or maybe confused by, what pulses are

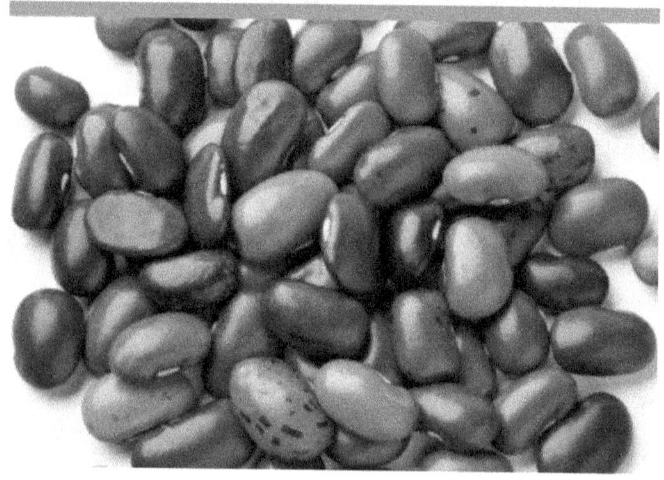

Give entire Foods Priority:

The foundation of your diet should consist of entire foods including fruits, vegetables, whole grains, lean meats, and healthy fats. These foods are abundant in fiber, antioxidants, and other nutrients that can promote general health, including breast health, and reduce inflammation. When eating, try to load up your plate with as many different colors of fruits and veggies as possible to guarantee you're getting a range of vitamins and minerals.

Read Labels and Avoid Hidden Sugars:

Even in items that don't taste sweet, hidden sugars are frequently present in processed foods. You can recognize and stay clear of these added sugars by learning to read food labels. Additive sugars are frequently found in ingredients such as dextrose, cane sugar, maltose, and high-fructose corn syrup. Choose items that are lower in sugar content and have fewer components. Moreover, goods tagged as "diet" or "low-fat" should also be avoided because they can have more added sugar to make up for the flavor.

Cook at Home:

When you cook at home, you can choose exactly what products you use and stay away from processed foods and added sugars that are frequently present in fast food and restaurant meals.
Instead of depending solely on premade sauces and condiments, try experimenting with straightforward recipes

that call for entire foods and a range of herbs and spices for taste. Cooking at home encourages better eating habits all around and helps lower consumption of manufactured foods.

Limit Packaged Snacks and Beverages:

Snacks in packages, such as cookies, candy bars, and chips, are frequently laden with artificial chemicals, harmful fats, and added sugars. Opt for more healthful snack alternatives like fresh fruit, yogurt, almonds, and seeds, or chopped veggies with nut butter or hummus.

Similarly, consuming too much sugar can be facilitated by sugary drinks such fruit juices, energy drinks, and soda. Choose homemade smoothies with natural sweeteners like fresh fruit or a small quantity of honey, or water or herbal tea.

Plan Ahead and Practice Moderation:

Arranging your meals and snacks in advance might assist you in choosing better options and preventing impulsive purchasing of processed foods. Make a whole-foods-based grocery list and follow it when you go grocery shopping.

Additionally, rather than starving yourself entirely, give yourself occasional delights in moderation. Occasionally indulging in small servings of your preferred processed foods can help quell cravings without unduly compromising your overall efforts to cut back on intake.

Limiting the intake of processed foods and added sugars can help prevent breast cancer and improve general health by taking preventative measures. You can drastically alter your diet and way of life by emphasizing whole foods, reading labels, cooking at home, selecting healthy snacks and drinks, and exercising sensibly. Recall that gradual improvements build up to a healthier, happier you, and that every healthy decision you make gets you one step closer to that goal.

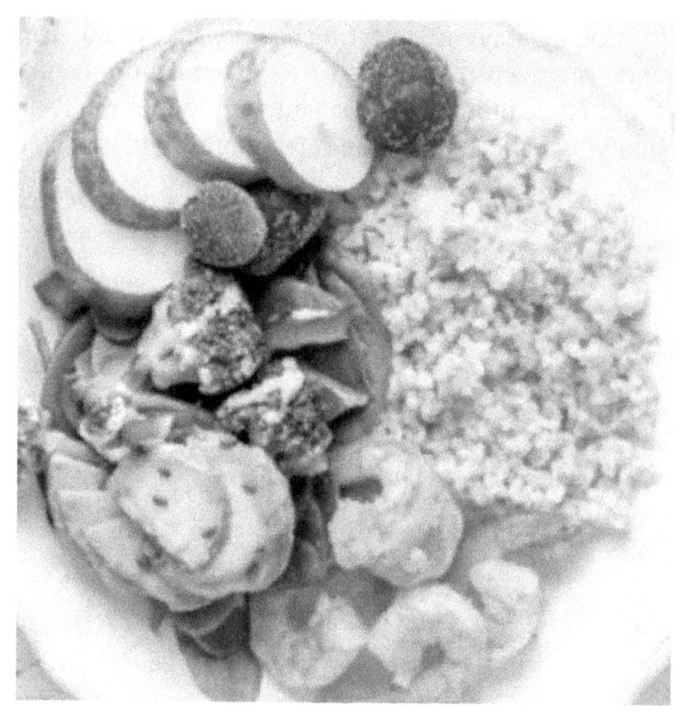

CHAPTER EIGHT

MAINTAINING A HEALTHY WEIGHT FOR BREAST CANCER PREVENTION

Exploring the Link Between Weight Management and Breast Cancer Risk

Research indicates a strong correlation between being overweight and a higher risk of breast cancer that develops after menopause. Visceral fat in particular functions as an active endocrine organ that can produce hormones like insulin, leptin, and estrogen—all of which are linked to the onset and spread of breast cancer. Increased levels of these hormones are linked to angiogenesis, inflammation, and cell proliferation—all of which are indicators of the spread of cancer.

Furthermore, a favorable milieu for the initiation and advancement of tumors is created by obesity, which is frequently associated with chronic low-grade inflammation. Adipokines, which are also produced by adipose tissue, have the ability to affect insulin resistance, a factor linked to an increased risk of breast cancer.

On the other hand, there is substantial evidence that weight control strategies, such as dietary adjustments, increased physical activity, and behavioral adjustments, can lower the risk of breast cancer. In addition to helping people lose weight, calorie restriction and a diet high in fruits, vegetables, whole grains, and lean meats also reduce inflammation and enhance metabolic health, which lowers the risk of breast cancer.

The Role of Hormonal Factors:

The primary hormone responsible for the development of breast cancer in premenopausal women is estrogen, which is produced by the ovaries. Adipocyte-produced excess estrogen can cause cancer, especially in postmenopausal women whose primary source of estrogen switches from the ovaries to adipose tissue. Lowering circulating estrogen levels and maintaining a healthy weight can lessen the risk of breast cancer.

Moreover, insulin resistance—which is frequently linked to obesity—promotes the synthesis of insulin-like growth factors (IGFs), which limit apoptosis and encourage cell division. Through weight management and lifestyle improvements aimed at enhancing insulin sensitivity, individuals may be able to reduce the risk of breast cancer caused by IGFs.

The Impact of Lifestyle Choices:

Beyond maintaining a healthy weight, lifestyle choices like alcohol use and physical activity level have a big impact on breast cancer risk. Overindulgence in alcohol has long been associated with an increased risk of breast cancer, especially hormone receptor-positive subtypes.

On the other hand, frequent exercise improves immune system performance, decreases inflammation, and lowers circulating estrogen levels, all of which minimize the risk of breast cancer in addition to helping with weight control.

Stopping Breast Cancer Risk in Its Tracks:

Educating people about the connection between controlling weight and breast cancer risk is essential to halting the disease's progression. Breast cancer risk can be considerably decreased by promoting good lifestyle choices, such as eating a balanced diet, getting regular exercise, abstaining from alcohol, and reaching and maintaining a healthy weight.

In addition, healthcare professionals are essential in encouraging preventive actions and providing assistance to people who want to lower their risk of breast cancer by changing their lifestyle. Healthcare practitioners can support early intervention and better patient outcomes by introducing weight management and its effect on breast cancer risk into regular clinical practice.

Results showed that Taking a comprehensive approach to cancer prevention is crucial, as seen by the link between breast cancer risk and weight management. Individuals can lower their risk of breast cancer by adopting proactive lifestyle alterations to address modifiable risk factors, such as excess weight.

We may work toward a day where breast cancer incidence is greatly reduced and lives are saved by well-informed decisions and focused interventions by continuing research, educating the public, and advocating for change.

Strategies for Achieving and Maintaining a Healthy Weight Through Diet

For many women, breast cancer is a constant worry, and one of the most important ways to avoid it is through lifestyle choices. Breast cancer risk is influenced by a variety of factors, including genetics, but eating a healthy weight can greatly lower the chance of getting the disease. With an emphasis on reducing the risk of breast cancer, we'll look at practical methods for reaching and maintaining a healthy weight through food choices in this book.

Accept a Diet Based on Plants:

Make sure your meals contain an abundance of fruits, veggies, whole grains, and legumes. These foods are high in phytochemicals, which have potent antioxidant qualities and help fight free radicals that cause cancer. They are also high in vitamins, minerals, fiber, and other nutrients.

Aim for a colorful plate since varied hues of fruits and vegetables provide a range of nutrients that support general health and lower the risk of cancer.

Restrict Red and Processed Meats:

Preservatives and additives found in processed meats like sausages, bacon, and deli meats have been connected to a higher risk of breast cancer. Consumption of red meat should also be kept in check.

Lean protein options include fish, poultry, tofu, tempeh, and lentils. These substitutes offer vital nutrients without the dangerous chemicals and saturated fats seen in processed meats.

Choose Healthy Fats:

Increase your intake of foods like avocados, almonds, seeds, and olive oil that are high in healthy fats. When ingested in moderation, these fats promote general health and can help with weight management.

Reduce your intake of the saturated and trans fats in fried foods, pastries, and processed snacks since they raise your risk of cancer by causing inflammation and weight gain.

Practice Portion Control:

Pay attention to portion sizes to avoid overindulging, which can result in weight gain. Eat mindfully, use smaller plates, and pay attention to your body's hunger signals. Aim to fill half of your plate with vegetables, one-quarter with lean protein, and one-quarter with healthy grains or starchy vegetables. Pay attention to the portion amounts suggested by nutrition labels.

Drink Water to Remain Hydrated:

To stay hydrated and avoid consuming extra calories from sugary drinks like soda and fruit juices, make water your main beverage choice.

Water consumption in moderation aids in appetite control, aids in digestion, and supports weight loss initiatives.

Prioritize Whole Foods:

Reduce your intake of refined and processed foods that are heavy in sugar, salt, and bad fats. These meals can cause inflammation and weight gain, and they have minimal nutritious benefit.

Choose whole, nutrient-dense foods to fuel your body and promote general well-being.

Pay Attention to Your Alcohol Consumption:

Limit your alcohol intake because drinking too much of it raises your chance of breast cancer. If you do decide to drink, try to limit your intake and once in a while choose red wine instead of white, as red wine has antioxidants like resveratrol.

Try to adhere to national recommendations for moderate alcohol intake, which generally suggest no more than one drink per day for women.

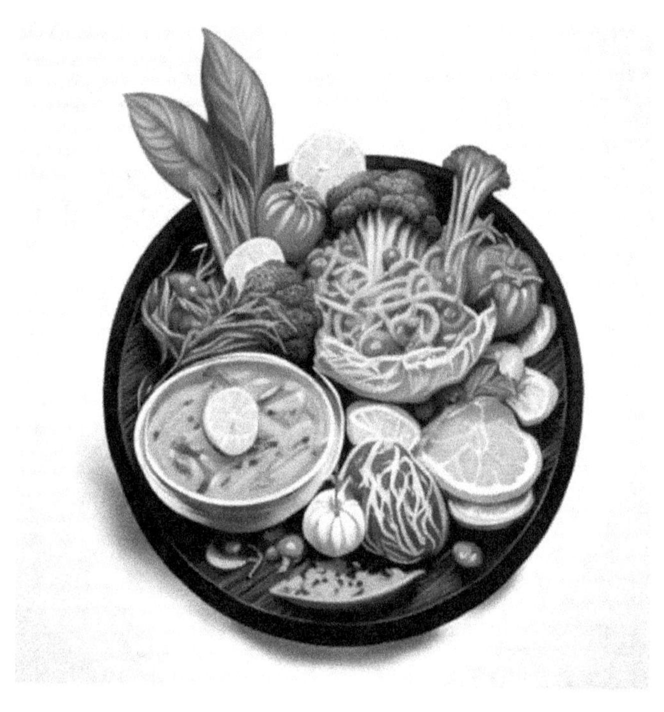

CHAPTER NINE

ALCOHOL CONSUMPTION AND BREAST CANCER RISK

Understanding The Connection Between Alcohol Consumption and Breast Cancer

There is unmistakable evidence from numerous studies linking alcohol use to a higher risk of breast cancer. The danger increases as alcohol use grows. It has been demonstrated that even moderate alcohol use increases the risk of breast cancer.

The body's metabolism of alcohol is the mechanism underlying this relationship. Acetaldehyde, a carcinogenic substance that can damage DNA and interfere with cell function and perhaps cause the creation of malignant cells, is produced when alcohol is digested.

Additionally, drinking alcohol can alter the body's levels of hormones, especially estrogen, which is vital for the development of breast cancer. Breast cancer risk has been associated with elevated estrogen levels, and alcohol use can exacerbate this imbalance. Alcohol may also make it more difficult for the body to absorb antioxidants and other vital nutrients, which raises the risk of cancer.

Stopping Breast Cancer Risk:

The good news is that there is a considerable reduction in the risk of breast cancer when alcohol usage is reduced or eliminated. Reducing alcohol use, even slightly, can improve general health and wellbeing. Here are some tactics to think about:

Education and Awareness: It's important to raise awareness of the connection between drinking alcohol and the risk of breast cancer. Making people aware of the possible effects of alcohol use on breast health, particularly women, can enable them to make more educated decisions about their lifestyles.

Moderation or Abstinence: Moderation is crucial for alcohol users who choose this decision. Reducing alcohol consumption to one drink per day for women will help lower their chance of developing breast cancer. On the other hand, the best strategy to remove this risk factor is to completely give up alcohol.

Healthy Lifestyle Options: Keeping a healthy weight, engaging in regular exercise, and eating a balanced diet high in fruits and vegetables can all help lower the risk of breast cancer. Additionally, these lifestyle choices can improve general health and wellbeing.

Frequent Screening: As advised by medical experts, women should have routine breast cancer screenings. Treatment results and survival rates can be greatly enhanced by early detection through screenings like mammography.

In our opinion, there is a complicated but important relationship between alcohol use and the risk of breast cancer in women.

People can lessen their chance of breast cancer and improve their general health by being aware of this link and taking proactive steps to cut back on alcohol use. Educating women and encouraging healthy lifestyle choices are critical components of the breast cancer prevention strategy.

Guidelines for Moderate Alcohol Consumption and Alternatives

Recognize Your Limits: For women, moderate alcohol consumption is usually described as no more than one drink per day. Knowing what a standard drink is is important because it usually has 14 grams of pure alcohol in it. Twelve ounces of beer, five ounces of wine, or 1.5 ounces of distilled spirits are a few examples.

Avoid drinking too much at once and spread out your alcoholic drinks over time. Drinking a lot of alcohol in a short amount of time can greatly raise the risk of breast cancer. Choose smaller portions and pair them with non-alcoholic drinks like juice or water.

Be Aware of Frequency: Frequency counts, even when drinking in moderation. Even moderate alcohol consumption on a regular basis may raise the risk of breast cancer. To give your body a vacation, think about designating some days of the week as alcohol-free.

Keep an Eye on quantity proportions: When pouring drinks at home, in particular, be mindful of quantity proportions. Over pouring may cause accidental overflow of advised volumes. Stick to the single servings offered at social occasions or use measuring instruments.

Think About Individual Factors: The relationship between alcohol and breast cancer risk can vary depending on a person's age, hormone levels, genetics, and general health. Speak with medical experts, particularly if you have other risk factors or a family history of breast cancer.

Alternatives to Drinking Alcohol:

Discover the world of non-alcoholic beverages and mocktails. Without the use of alcohol, several recipes provide rich flavors and possibilities for refreshing drinks. Try creating pleasing substitutes by experimenting with components such as flavored syrups, fresh fruits, and herbs.

Herbal Teas: As an alternative to alcoholic beverages, herbal teas are calming and reassuring. Herbal mixes come in a variety of tastes and may have various health advantages, including soothing properties and antioxidants. Relax with a warm cup of herbal tea as a bedtime ritual.

Sparkling Water: A effervescent and cool substitute for alcoholic beverages is sparkling water that has been naturally flavored. Sparkling water is a pleasant substitute for alcoholic beverages at social gatherings. It comes in a variety of flavors, from citrus to berry.

Fruit Infused Water: To enhance flavor and aesthetic appeal, infuse water with slices of fruits, vegetables, or herbs. Make your own blends, like strawberry and basil or cucumber and mint. Fruit-infused water provides a natural flavor boost and moisturizes the body.

Wellness Activities: As an alternative to drinking alcohol, partake in wellness activities that encourage stress relief and relaxation. Without the use of alcohol, techniques like yoga, meditation, and deep breathing exercises can help reduce stress and enhance general wellbeing.

In conclusion, it's important to understand how moderate alcohol use may affect the risk of breast cancer, even though it's a personal decision. By following moderation rules and considering other options, people can make well-informed decisions that put their health and wellbeing first.

Incorporating healthy lifestyle choices and seeking medical advice can bolster initiatives to reduce the risk of breast cancer and enhance general wellness.

Healthy Recipe: Quinoa Breakfast Porridge

Feel free to use any topping you'd like

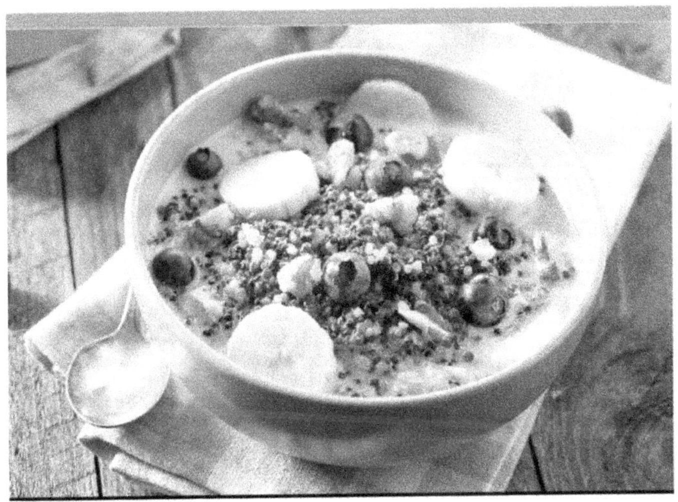

CHAPTER TEN

CREATING A BREAST CANCER PREVENTION MEAL PLAN

Practical Tips for Planning and Preparing Meals That Support Breast Health

Meal planning for breast health involves a number of things, such as adding foods high in nutrients that are known to benefit breast health, keeping a balanced diet, and reducing the use of substances that may raise the risk of breast cancer. The following useful advice can be used to organize and prepare meals that fully support breast health:

Include a range of fruits and veggies: Try to make your meals consist of a vibrant assortment of fruits and vegetables. Antioxidants, vitamins, minerals, and fiber-rich diets can help lower inflammation and promote general breast health. Add cruciferous vegetables to your diet, such as Brussels sprouts, kale, and broccoli, as they contain substances that may help lower your chance of developing breast cancer.

Select lean protein sources: Tofu, fish, poultry, lentils, and beans are examples of lean protein sources. Iron and protein, two important minerals, are provided by these foods without the additional saturated fat that comes with red meat.

Add sources of healthy fats to your diet: Avocados, nuts, seeds, and olive oil are a few examples of foods high in healthy fats. These fats may help lower the risk of breast cancer because they contain molecules with anti-inflammatory qualities, such as omega-3 fatty acids.

Limit saturated and trans fats: Reduce your intake of foods high in trans and saturated fats, such as processed meats, fried foods, and commercially baked pastries. An elevated risk of breast cancer and other health problems has been linked to these lipids.

Choose whole grains: Rather than refined grains, choose whole grains like brown rice, quinoa, oats, and whole wheat bread. Whole grains are high in fiber, vitamins, and minerals, which can support overall health and lower the risk of breast cancer.

Limit added sugars: Eat fewer foods and drinks high in added sugars, such as sodas, sugary snacks, and sweets. Consuming a lot of sugar has been linked to insulin resistance and obesity, two conditions that increase the risk of breast cancer.

Include foods rich in phytoestrogens: These plant compounds, which mimic the effects of estrogen in the body, such as soy products, flaxseeds, and legumes, in your diet. These foods may help regulate estrogen levels and lower the

Stay hydrated: Keep yourself hydrated by sipping on lots of water throughout the day. Restrict your intake of alcohol and sugary drinks because drinking too much of it has been related to a higher risk of breast cancer.

Use portion control: Pay attention to serving sizes to prevent overindulging, which raises the risk of breast cancer and contributes to weight gain. Measure portion sizes, use smaller plates, and pay attention to your body's signals of hunger and fullness.

Make a plan and cook at home: Making a plan and cooking at home gives you more control over the ingredients and cooking techniques you utilize. Try preparing more meals from scratch using whole, fresh ingredients and consuming fewer packaged and processed foods.

Seek professional advice: You should think about speaking with a qualified dietitian or nutritionist if you have any specific dietary questions or medical conditions, such as breast cancer or a family history of the disease. They can offer you individualized guidance and assistance in optimizing your diet for breast health.

You may significantly improve breast health and lower your chance of developing breast cancer by implementing these useful recommendations into the planning and preparation of your meals. Always remember to seek for balance, diversity, and moderation in your diet, and to concentrate on general dietary patterns rather than specific foods or substances.

Sample meal plans and recipes for a balanced and nutritious diet

In terms of nutrition and breast cancer, maintaining general health and maybe lowering the chance of recurrence can be greatly aided by eating a balanced, nutrient-rich diet. Here is an example meal plan with recipes that emphasize consuming foods high in vitamins, minerals, antioxidants, and healthy fats—all of which are good for those who have breast cancer:

Breakfast:
Avocado and Spinach Omelette:

Ingredients:

2 eggs

1/4 cup chopped spinach

1/4 avocado, sliced

Salt and pepper to taste

Instructions:

Add salt and pepper to a dish of beaten eggs. Place the beaten eggs into a nonstick skillet and cook it over medium heat.

Place the avocado slices and chopped spinach on one half of the omelette once the eggs begin to set.
After folding the other half over the filling, fry the eggs until they are completely set. Warm up and serve.

Mixed Berry Smoothie:

Ingredients:

Half cup of berries blended together with strawberries, blueberries, and raspberries

Half banana, half a cup of spinach

A quarter of a cup Greek yogurt

One-half cup almond milk

If preferred, one teaspoon of honey

Instructions:

Combine all ingredients in a blender and blend until smooth. Add more almond milk if needed to reach desired consistency. Serve immediately.

Mid-Morning Snack:
Greek Yogurt with Almonds and Berries:

Ingredients:

A quarter of a cup Greek yogurt
1/4 cup of mixed berries (blueberries, raspberries)
A single spoonful of sliced almonds
If preferred, one tsp honey

Instructions:

Place Greek yogurt in a bowl and top with mixed berries and sliced almonds.

Drizzle with honey if desired. Enjoy!

Lunch:
Grilled Salmon Salad:

Ingredients:

A 4-oz grilled salmon fillet
two glasses of mixed greens salad
1/4 cup chopped cherry tomatoes 1/4 sliced cucumber 1/4 of an avocado, cut into slices
One tablespoon of olive oil by itself

One-third cup balsamic vinegar
To taste, add more salt and pepper.

Instructions:

On a serving platter, arrange the avocado, cherry tomatoes, cucumber, and mixed salad greens.
Top with grilled salmon.
To make the dressing, combine the olive oil, balsamic vinegar, salt, and pepper in a small bowl.
After dressing the salad, drizzle over it and serve.

Afternoon Snack:
Carrot Sticks with Hummus:

Ingredients:

1 medium carrot, cut into sticks

2 tablespoons hummus

Instructions:

Serve carrot sticks with hummus for dipping.

Dinner:
Quinoa-Stuffed Bell Peppers:

Ingredients:

Two large bell peppers, cut in half and seedless
One-half cup of cooked quinoa
A half-cup of rinsed and drained black beans
One-half cup of kernel corn
a quarter cup finely sliced tomatoes
1/4 cup of red onion, thinly sliced
One-fourth cup of shredded cheese
A single tsp of hot sauce
Half a teaspoon of cumin
To taste, add more salt and pepper.

Instructions:

Roast at 190°C, or 375°F, in the oven.
Cooked quinoa, black beans, corn, tomatoes, red onion,
shredded cheese, cumin, chili powder, salt, and pepper
should all be combined in a bowl.
Stuff the inside of the bell peppers with the quinoa mixture
on all sides.
After putting the filled peppers on a baking sheet, bake
them for 25 to 30 minutes, or until the filling is thoroughly
heated and the peppers are soft.
Warm up the food.

Evening Snack:
Whole Grain Crackers with Sliced Cheese:

Ingredients:

Whole grain crackers

Sliced cheese (such as cheddar or Swiss)

Instructions:

Serve whole grain crackers with sliced cheese for a satisfying snack.

A range of nutrient-dense foods are included in this meal plan to enhance general health and wellbeing both before and after breast cancer treatment. It minimizes processed meals and added sweets while consuming an abundance of fruits, vegetables, whole grains, lean protein, and healthy fats.

Don't forget to adjust ingredients and portions to suit specific dietary requirements and personal preferences. For individualized dietary advice, it's also critical to speak with a medical professional or certified dietitian.

CONCLUSION

In summary, the "Stopping Breast Cancer Cookbook Guide" provides a plan to empower people on their path to breast health in addition to a plethora of nutritional meals. By combining scientific knowledge with culinary know-how, this guide highlights the significant influence of nutrition on managing and preventing breast cancer.

Let us take with us the knowledge that every meal we prepare is an opportunity to strengthen our bodies against illness as we close the pages of this book. Accept the idea that food serves as more than just nourishment—rather, it can be an effective weapon in our fight against breast cancer.

I hope that this cookbook will be a source of inspiration and guidance as we move toward a time when fewer people are diagnosed with breast cancer and everyone is aware of how to protect their own health. With the help of the delectable and nourishing recipes included in these pages, let's set off on a journey toward health and vitality together.

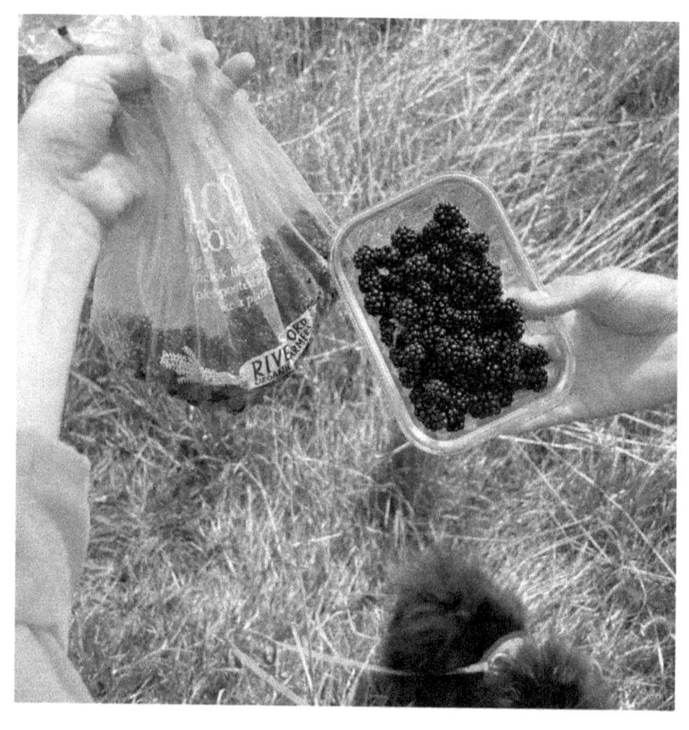

BONUS

7-DAY MEAL PLAN DESIGNED FOR BREAST CANCER

Certainly! Here's a sample 7-day meal plan designed to support breast health for women over 40. This plan focuses on incorporating foods rich in antioxidants, fiber, and healthy fats, which are beneficial for overall well-being and may help reduce the risk of breast cancer:

Day 1:

Breakfast:

Greek yogurt topped with fresh berries and a sprinkle of chia seeds.

Whole grain toast with avocado slices.

Lunch:

Grilled chicken salad with mixed greens, tomatoes, cucumbers, and olive oil vinaigrette.

A side of quinoa salad with diced vegetables.

Dinner:

Baked salmon seasoned with herbs and lemon juice.

Steamed broccoli and carrots.

Quinoa pilaf with spinach and almonds.

Snack:

A small handful of mixed nuts (such as almonds, walnuts, and pistachios).

Carrot sticks with hummus.

Day 2:

Breakfast:

Oatmeal topped with sliced bananas and a drizzle of honey.

A glass of almond milk.

Lunch:

Whole grain wrap filled with grilled vegetables and hummus.

A side of kale salad with cranberries and pumpkin seeds.

Dinner:

Turkey meatballs served with whole wheat pasta and marinara sauce.

Steamed green beans.

Mixed berry salad with a balsamic glaze.

Snack:

Plain Greek yogurt with a spoonful of almond butter.

Sliced apple.

Day 3:

Breakfast:

Whole grain toast topped with mashed avocado and sliced tomatoes.

Scrambled eggs with spinach and bell peppers.

Lunch:

Quinoa and black bean salad with diced avocado and lime vinaigrette.

A side of roasted sweet potatoes.

Dinner:

Grilled shrimp skewers with pineapple chunks and bell peppers.

Brown rice pilaf with mixed herbs.

Steamed asparagus spears.

Snack:

Cottage cheese with pineapple chunks.

Whole grain crackers with sliced cucumber.

Day 4:

Breakfast:

Smoothie made with spinach, kale, banana, almond milk, and a scoop of protein powder.

Whole grain toast with almond butter.

Lunch:

Vegetable stir-fry with tofu served over brown rice.

Side of edamame beans.

Dinner:

Baked chicken breast with rosemary and garlic.

Roasted Brussels sprouts with balsamic glaze.

Quinoa and vegetable medley.

Snack:

Trail mix with dried cranberries, almonds, and pumpkin seeds.

Celery sticks with peanut butter.

Day 5:
Breakfast:
Whole grain pancakes topped with mixed berries and a drizzle of maple syrup.

A glass of orange juice.

Lunch:
Spinach and strawberry salad with grilled chicken breast and balsamic vinaigrette.

A side of whole grain roll.

Dinner:
Baked cod fillets with lemon and herbs.

Sautéed spinach with garlic.

Whole grain couscous with diced vegetables.

Snack:
Low-fat string cheese.

Grapes.

Day 6:

Breakfast:

Vegetable omelet with mushrooms, onions, and bell peppers.

Whole grain toast with avocado spread.

Lunch:

Quinoa and black bean stuffed bell peppers.

Side of mixed green salad with lemon-tahini dressing.

Dinner:

Grilled tofu skewers with teriyaki sauce.

Stir-fried vegetables with sesame seeds.

Brown rice.

Snack:

Plain Greek yogurt with sliced peaches.

Whole grain crackers with cheese.

Day 7:

Breakfast:

Chia seed pudding topped with sliced almonds and fresh berries.

A side of whole grain toast with almond butter.

Lunch:

Mediterranean chickpea salad with feta cheese, cherry tomatoes, and olives.

A side of whole grain pita bread.

Dinner:

Baked tilapia with a mango salsa topping.

Steamed broccoli and cauliflower.

Quinoa salad with diced cucumber and mint.

Snack:

Air-popped popcorn sprinkled with nutritional yeast.

Sliced bell peppers with hummus.

Remember to drink plenty of water throughout the day and adjust portion sizes according to individual calorie needs.

Additionally, it's essential to consult with a healthcare professional or a registered dietitian before making significant changes to your diet, especially if you have specific health concerns or dietary restrictions.

EXERCISE PROGRAM INCORPORATED

Exercise and Its Impact on Breast Cancer: Understanding Types and Benefits

Exercise plays a crucial role in maintaining overall health and well-being, and it can be particularly beneficial for individuals affected by breast cancer. Engaging in regular physical activity not only helps improve physical fitness but also contributes to emotional well-being and quality of life during and after cancer treatment. Understanding the different types of exercises and their benefits can empower individuals to incorporate suitable activities into their lifestyle.

Types of Exercise:

Aerobic Exercise: Also known as cardio, aerobic exercise involves activities that increase the heart rate and breathing rate. These include brisk walking, jogging, cycling, swimming, and dancing. Aerobic exercise helps improve cardiovascular health, endurance, and overall fitness. It also promotes weight management and may reduce the risk of cancer recurrence.

Strength Training: Strength training involves exercises that target specific muscle groups using resistance, such as weights, resistance bands, or bodyweight exercises like push-ups and squats. Building strength helps maintain muscle mass, bone density, and functional capacity. It also aids in managing treatment-related side effects like fatigue and muscle weakness.

Flexibility and Stretching: Flexibility exercises focus on improving joint mobility and range of motion. Stretching routines can include yoga, Pilates, and specific stretching exercises. These activities enhance flexibility, reduce muscle tension, and improve posture. They also promote relaxation and stress relief, which are essential for overall well-being.

Balance and Stability Training: Balance exercises help improve coordination and stability, reducing the risk of falls and injuries. These activities include standing on one leg, heel-to-toe walking, and balance board exercises. Enhancing balance and stability contributes to functional independence and confidence in daily activities.

Benefits of Exercise for Breast Cancer Patients and Survivors:

Improved Physical Function: Regular exercise can help alleviate treatment-related side effects such as fatigue, muscle weakness, and joint stiffness. It enhances physical function and restores energy levels, enabling individuals to better cope with daily tasks and activities.

Enhanced Emotional Well-being: Exercise has been shown to boost mood, reduce anxiety and depression, and improve overall psychological well-being. Physical activity releases endorphins, the body's natural mood lifters, promoting feelings of happiness and relaxation.

Reduced Risk of Recurrence: Studies suggest that engaging in regular exercise may lower the risk of breast cancer recurrence and improve long-term survival rates. Exercise helps regulate hormone levels, reduce inflammation, and support immune function, all of which contribute to a lower risk of cancer progression.

Supportive Community and Social Connection:

Participating in group exercise classes or joining support groups for cancer survivors fosters a sense of community and social connection. Sharing experiences and engaging in activities with others who understand can provide valuable emotional support and encouragement.

Empowerment and Control: Taking an active role in one's health through exercise empowers individuals and instills a sense of control over their bodies. Setting and achieving fitness goals, overcoming challenges, and experiencing improvements in physical fitness contribute to a positive outlook and sense of accomplishment.

Safety Considerations:

Before starting any exercise program, it's essential for individuals affected by breast cancer to consult with their healthcare team, particularly if they have undergone surgery or are undergoing treatment. Here are some safety considerations:

Gradually increase the intensity and duration of exercise to avoid overexertion.

Listen to your body and adjust the level of activity based on how you feel.

Use proper form and technique to prevent injuries, especially during strength training.

Stay hydrated and take breaks as needed, especially in hot weather.

Wear appropriate clothing and supportive footwear to ensure comfort and safety during exercise.

In conclusion, exercise plays a vital role in supporting the physical and emotional well-being of individuals affected by breast cancer. By incorporating a variety of exercises into their routine, individuals can improve their overall health, manage treatment-related side effects, and enhance their quality of life during and after cancer treatment.

With guidance from healthcare professionals and support from peers, exercise becomes a powerful tool for empowerment and resilience on the journey to recovery and survivorship.

HAPPY READING!!